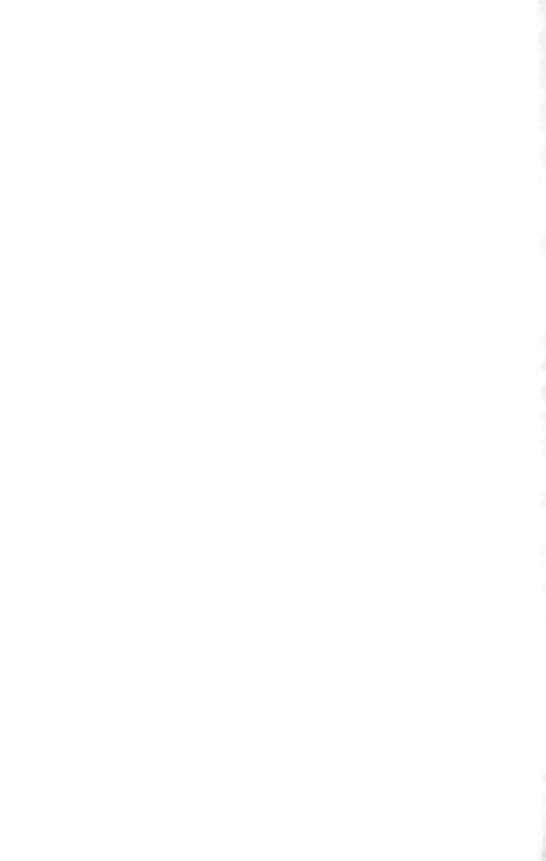

# The
# Dental Assisting
# Handbook

## A How-to Guide for
## Confidence and Success

Robert E. Porter, DDS

ISBN:   978-1-963569-69-8  (Hard Cover)
        978-1-963569-70-4  (Soft Cover)

Porter. Robert.

Edited by: Melissa Long
Photos by Carina Teleha, Carina Studios

Published by Warren Publishing
Charlotte, NC
www.warrenpublishing.net
Printed in the United States

*I dedicate this book to my children.*

# Acknowledgments

I want to thank the devoted editors at Warren Publishing whose partnership allowed my vision for this book to become a reality. I owe tremendous gratitude to my family and colleagues for their steadfast support and thoughtful contributions. I want to thank my father, Dr. Charles Porter III, for sharing invaluable lessons from his years of experience as a dentist. His collaboration has positively shaped this text from the first written words to the last. Many thanks to my mother whose keen eyes kept my writing clear and consistent. Thank you to my sister, Dr. Rebecca Wilson, who assisted with clinical photography and ensured the visuals were captivating and engaging. Thank you to Dr. William Wilson and Dr. Richard Chu for their careful reviews and insights, and whose sage advice always reflected concern for future readers. As always, thank you to my loving wife for her constant support in all my endeavors. I am forever grateful for the dentists before me whose persistence and dedication carved a path to better dentistry, and to the many unsung dental assistants who provided steadfast care every step of the way.

# Preface

Dental assisting is a truly unique career path that provides limitless opportunities for personal and professional growth. Positive career trajectory and momentum in the field of dental assisting largely depends on mastery of communication, clinical skills, and a broad understanding of the dental profession. Many qualities of high-performing dental assistants and steps for complex dental procedures can be learned by implementing simple, repeatable behaviors. There really is a recipe for success, and motivated individuals deserve a resource that effectively outlines these behavioral skills for people of all levels of dental-assisting experience in a simple format designed to advance careers.

With routine practice, dedication, and trusted educational resources, anyone can achieve a high level of success as an integral member of a dental team. This text is a proven guide created by dentists to provide the foundational concepts of dentistry, common workplace expectations, and effective professional behaviors for dental assisting. This information will empower prospective dental assistants with knowledge and confidence as proven behaviors are taught and reinforced to exceed work expectations and achieve fulfilling careers. So, meet the doctors who will guide you through your first dental assisting handbook, and learn why they designed this resource specifically for you.

Dr. Charles and Dr. Robert Porter are father-and-son general dentists with over thirty years of combined experience. They are continuously adapting to new dental materials and technologies, and leading a skilled team with the mission to provide the best dental care possible. Their family-owned dental practice, Porter Dental Group, is located in Charlotte, North Carolina where they strive to provide every patient with excellent, personalized care. At the heart of their dental practice is a team of dedicated dental assistants whose work ethic, commitment, and conscientious care help craft wonderful doctor-patient experiences.

Dr. Charles and Dr. Robert believe personal attention is the key to cultivating positive, relaxed patient care in a profession stigmatized by daunting, uncomfortable procedures. Having the most up-to-date dental office matters little if patients do not feel human concern and compassion for their health and well-being. Dental offices can be equipped with the newest dental technologies and best dental materials for quality dentistry, but if providers of these resources fail to convey genuine care, patients will not recognize and experience the value of exceptional dentistry. In order to maintain a first-class atmosphere, all administrative staff and dental-care providers must be confident, well-trained, and knowledgeable about their respective roles so patients feel cared for in every aspect of their dental visits.

Dental assistants are core, essential team members at a dental office as they spend most of their time chairside. The quality of interactions alongside patients can largely impact how those patients perceive the quality of their dental care regardless of how procedures are technically performed. Professional interactions and relationships are critical and will determine the success of the practice.

Historically, many dental assistants entered the workforce with minimal formal training on behaviors and communication techniques that foster professionalism and promote productive teamwork. A lack of education for these successful occupational behaviors led to persistent deficits in preparedness for dental assistants entering the workforce.

The minimal development of these soft skills was worsened by the COVID-19 pandemic.

In 2020, due to the dangers of COVID-19, most schools and training programs sent students home to learn remotely. The pandemic had devastating health consequences for many and lasting impacts for nearly every business. Both patients and healthcare providers experienced uncertainty with in-person care, as basic medical supplies were limited, and the status of community-spread infection was unknown. Students enrolled in healthcare training programs relying on face-to-face instruction experienced tremendous hardships as they lost opportunities to develop and hone clinical skills.

Many programs transitioned to online platforms, streaming content without personalized reinforcement. This change reshaped student experience and learning outcomes. The minimal dental-assistant training provided pre-COVID-19 for communication and professionalism was further diminished, as students failed to receive the interpersonal feedback from in-person training. Educational institutions are still rebounding from this monumental event in history. The effects of prolonged disruption to student learning are still seen as new graduates enter the workforce with career expectations and aspirations hindered by inconsistent education.

Without new resources, Dr. Charles and Dr. Robert wholeheartedly believe dental assistants will continue to face significant professional limitations, and the dental profession will suffer. So, new resources must emerge to support, equip, and promote dental assistants to be fully capable of facing all workforce challenges with knowledge, skills, and professionalism for the success they deserve.

Dr. Charles and Dr. Robert dedicated themselves to developing this curriculum of written lessons organized for new and prospective dental assistants to help bridge the gap from personal learning and introductory coursework to working hands-on in dental offices. These doctors recognized common hardships new dental assistants routinely faced and have compiled extensive lessons to prepare dental assistants for common clinical scenarios, prioritizing office duties, and problem-solving in the dental profession. Dental assistants deserve resources to make the transition from education to work predictable, so this straightforward guide was established with specific behaviors to launch and advance successful professional careers.

These lessons have been reviewed by dentists who are deeply committed to maintaining the quality and integrity of the dental profession and wish to promote and support the education of dental assistants. Porter Dental Group extends its heartfelt gratitude to all parties who invested time and energy to make this resource informative and impactful. We hope this text serves as a helpful reference for anyone interested in a career in chairside assisting or who wishes to learn more about this valued and cherished profession. We want all dental assistants to feel the confidence and satisfaction of helping provide excellent service for patients. With initiative, motivation, and the proper training, dental assisting can be the start to endless opportunities.

# Introduction

Acareer in dental assisting can provide a wealth of opportunities to interact with new people, render much-needed health services, and sustain an interesting and fulfilling work environment. For a profession that offers so much, there are few resources that provide an in-depth look at how to begin this role, develop a wide scope of techniques for professional success, and face routine challenges with confidence. This handbook will provide a personal roadmap for anyone interested in expanding professional horizons and navigating common career challenges in dental assisting as clinical knowledge and professional competency flourishes.

Dental assistants are integral team members, as they allow for smooth provision of complex procedures and help balance the busyness of a dental practice with efficiency. When dental assisting is performed well, patients can experience faster and more comfortable dentistry. Improved efficiency also allows the practice to meet overhead expenses, like paying for materials, new equipment, and staff wages and raises. The job security and stability of an excellent dental assistant is unmatched. To become a highly valued dental assistant, the journey starts with building a basic understanding of the profession.

There is an abundance of information available about nearly every career imaginable, and it can be overwhelming to wade through facts and opinions to uncover clear, honest information. Navigating a path to success in dental assisting can be confusing when so many resources conflict. So, practicing dentists have collaborated to create this universal guide to teach the fundamentals of general dentistry and dental assisting. There are many nuances to using dental materials and following the proper sequence of dental procedures. Dental assistants deserve credible, organized, dentist-approved resources to apply the emotional and technical training important to clinical dentistry.

There is no substitution for in-person education and training for hands-on careers. However, this reference will provide the prerequisite knowledge expected of all dental assistants prior to firsthand experiences. If you are considering or have already committed to paying the thousands of dollars to enroll in a dental assisting program, we want you to reap the most from your investment. This resource will strengthen your understanding of dental assisting before, during, and after completion of any dental assisting course, as you become fully aware of common job expectations and further cultivate the skills necessary to meet them with confidence. This resource will also help administrative team members in a dental office to better communicate aspects of dental procedures to patients, as well as cross-train these individuals in the event that additional clinical assistance is needed.

Even if you choose not to continue reading, please take time to learn the possible challenges and rewards of dental assisting before committing to a paid course. Transitioning to a new job can be challenging. So, avoid unwarranted stress by establishing realistic expectations, and empower yourself with knowledge of your future role. Every dental assistant deserves opportunities to be successful and confident in their careers.

# What Is Dental Assisting?

Many patients go to dental offices to have their teeth checked, cleaned, or repaired. Patients typically have their teeth cleaned by *dental hygienists*, and a dentist will oversee patients during a brief portion of the visit. A dental hygienist will often work one-on-one with patients, clean teeth, teach oral hygiene, and take dental X-rays. If patients have decayed, broken, or painful teeth, they will likely be seen exclusively by a dentist and a dental assistant.

*Dental assisting* is a job in the field of dentistry that involves working alongside dentists to provide dental treatment. The most common job duties for dental assistants are arranging materials for dental procedures and handing instruments and supplies directly to the doctor while treatment is performed. Dental assistants allow dentistry to be provided more efficiently and effectively by delivering what is needed directly into the dentist's hands during treatment and helping keep the patient's cheeks, lips, and tongue protected while treatment is performed. The term *Four-handed Dentistry* refers to dental procedures involving dentists and assistants working simultaneously, four hands in harmony.

Some other common duties for dental assistants include taking dental X-rays; assessing inventory of supplies before, during, and after dental procedures; and communicating with patients and coworkers to plan future appointments. A few common dental procedures that often involve a dental assistant include fillings, crowns, root canals, extractions, and impressions. More information about these specific procedures will be explained in detail later.

Dental assistants have physical, hands-on jobs and spend much of the workday standing or moving. This aspect of dental assisting is very appealing to individuals who want careers that involve movement and are not limited to the confines of a desk. Dental assistants also work with multiple people every day, many of whom are anxious or in pain. Successful assistants have calm demeanors and are outgoing. Shy personalities can flourish in dental assisting roles as long as patients receive thoughtful attention.

Attention to detail with clinical procedures and a broad understanding of dentistry are very important. Many aspects of dentistry can be learned, but you must first have an awareness of your own strengths and weaknesses to recognize if you can meet the daily challenges of clinical dentistry. If you are searching for a job that allows you to move throughout the day, interact with other people, and test your mental agility with anticipating and navigating change, dental assisting may be a good fit for you.

# Qualities of Happy Assistants

Dental assistants have unique job roles that often benefit from a blend of different personality traits. Of the many traits complementing the profession, attentiveness to detail, organization skills, and anticipation skills are most important. Dentistry involves repetition and following a very specific sequence of steps with corresponding instruments and materials. It can be compared to a dance—procedural steps must flow eloquently in rhythm and sequence.

Personal energy is the catalyst that allows attention and organization to be useful for performing procedures efficiently. It is okay to have a reserved personality, but you must be motivated and energetic in how you operate so procedural steps can be executed with positive momentum. Energetic people are highly successful as dental assistants because they can quickly proceed to appropriate steps, shorten appointment times, and foster a positive clinical atmosphere. Patients recognize the amount of time they spend at a dental office, and reducing treatment times often reduces patient anxiety and hesitation with future treatment.

Attentiveness to detail is critical for success with every dental procedure. Failure to provide thoughtful care can result in patients receiving poor treatment that takes longer, is painful, and may not last over time. The sequence of steps in a procedure, exchange of instruments between doctor and assistant, and awareness of the patient's tissues all require careful attention and are important so the dental visit may be efficient and minimize patient discomfort.

Maintaining treatment room organization allows for ease of exchange of instruments and supplies. If instruments are in order throughout a procedure, they can be more easily identified and selected for delivery to the doctor, resulting in more efficient dentistry.

Anticipation will be expected throughout the day, especially during clinical procedures. Dental assistants must be thoughtfully engaged during dental treatment and constantly thinking about next steps so instruments and materials can be ready. Lapse in focus will delay treatment and could jeopardize treatment success.

No one starts a new job knowing exactly how to perform it as expected, but new dental assistants will be expected to quickly learn basic techniques and become familiar with a vast array of dental materials. Navigating new clinical experiences will require assistants to actively listen and closely follow instructions. After all, dental assistants work within a very personal space for patients, and with the patient's health and comfort at stake, there is little room for errors or mishaps. It is important not only to know what materials and instruments are required for each procedure, but to be able to quickly locate different materials in an office when procedures change mid-treatment.

Familiarize yourself with the supply inventory at your office so you can retrieve materials as needed. Even with the most diligent preparation, you will inevitably encounter changes in treatment you are unfamiliar with. Stay focused and receptive to guidance from the dentist as you navigate new clinical experiences.

For those new to the dental profession, there is a tremendous volume of new information to learn and apply, presenting a steep learning curve. But with commitment and dedication, you will soon become familiar with how procedures flow and what your dentist needs and expects. Ultimately, you will know every step in routine dental procedures and be able to provide the dentist with the necessary materials from start to finish, allowing appointments to flow smoothly.

You may find there is not much communication between an assistant and a dentist during a clinical procedure because the exchange of instruments is so well-anticipated and seamless. Communication with patients is very important to help assess discomfort levels and patient concerns during visits, but this level of verbal communication may not be necessary between the dentist and assistant for much of the dental procedure. If the procedure is well-anticipated, there may be little conversation amongst the clinical team. This may seem like a daunting task to execute for beginners. Remember, dental procedures are repetitive, so you will start to recognize similarities in how procedures are performed and patterns for what is expected.

As you begin your role as a dental assistant, do not be discouraged if you encounter many new clinical experiences with which you are unfamiliar. Dentistry is performed based on patients' needs and desires, and dental treatments can vary tremendously from day-to-day at a general dentistry practice. Do your best to learn from your new experiences and commit new skills to memory. With time, you will soon have a basic understanding of many dental procedures.

If you are uncertain of whether dental assisting is the right career path for you, that is okay. There are many other job opportunities in dentistry or healthcare you can explore. Knowledge of dental assisting will only promote your understanding of your personal oral health and provide you with a more distinguished skillset if you choose to transition to other roles in a dental office.

To summarize, here are some common character traits of happy dental assistants:

- Attentive
- Proactive
- Calm
- Outgoing
- Sympathetic

# Rewards

Dental assisting undoubtedly presents unique challenges, as every tooth and patient is different. However, each challenge is paired with a unique reward dental assistants may experience. Managing patients and navigating complex treatments will regularly test critical-thinking and problem-solving skills. Meeting a multitude of challenges in dental assisting will develop character traits and establish relationships, which will benefit assistants well beyond the hours spent at a dental office. You will also strengthen your communication skills, clinical dexterity, and dental health knowledge in this profession. The knowledge and experiences that accompany time and dedication to dental assisting will provide intrinsic and extrinsic rewards for a very prosperous future.

A lot of dental assistants find they have more confidence speaking with other people, and this confidence is fostered by a career with many one-on-one, personal interactions while providing much-needed health services. Assistants often build strong relationships by helping patients overcome treatment anxieties through encouragement and emotional support. Patients should never have their fears discredited, and assistants should recognize and validate the patients' emotions regarding dental treatment while also encouraging them to proceed with treatments that improve their dental health and well-being. This aspect of dental assisting requires coaching and practice. We've all had coaches in different facets of life who we've grown to respect and appreciate, and if assistants can successfully and gracefully guide patients through dental treatment, they, in turn may also be held in high esteem.

Dental assistants become well-versed in a wide array of dental procedures, and this knowledge can help protect their own dental health and the health of friends and family. Often, dentistry becomes urgent when patients fail to maintain their oral health consistently at home. Assistants are very knowledgeable about effective oral hygiene habits to prevent dental disease, and this knowledge can be easily shared to benefit relationships outside the workplace. Should dental needs arise, assistants are also familiar with conservative dental treatment options and a network of providers for quality dental care.

Dental assisting is a physical, hands-on job, and there are many health benefits of moving throughout the day and using hand-eye coordination. You will strengthen your core, arms, and hands with static and dynamic muscle activity, burning calories and maintaining muscle tone. You will also establish and strengthen social interactions, which is important for overall health, as the need for human connection is innately ingrained in human psychology. One of the most appreciated rewards of dental assisting is building an exciting career that starkly differs from the monotony of an administrative role.

This is also a career path that does not require lengthy education for certification, so career transitions can be made quickly if individuals are looking for a new change. The cost of education is relatively low, so a career can be started with minimal personal debt or investment. With consistency, there are many opportunities for advancement in pay and responsibilities. The biggest indicator for future success is the ability to become an integral team member.

To summarize, here are some common rewards of dental assisting:

- Confidence
- Dental Knowledge
- Movement
- Coordination
- Minimal education cost

# The Seven

**M**any characteristics of great team members are universal. Whether in the workplace or on a sports team, there are common character traits and behaviors that foster success when working with other people. Not every individual on a team must be a leader, but there must be common values so team members can rely on each other, work together cohesively, and achieve their goals.

Learning how to work well in a team is critical for success in most careers, especially dental assisting. Humans are not innately born with effective communication skills and work habits. These traits must be routinely exercised to maintain strong interpersonal skills. Fortunately, there is a recipe for success, and following certain steps and respecting key values will guide you to a predictable work life.

The following is a culmination of expectations every team member should follow to maintain a calm and effective work environment. Some of these expectations may seem simple. But just like in many recipes, it is the simple, wholesome ingredients that produce spectacular meals. And keep in mind that abiding by these principles may not always be easy. Just like with routine exercise, implementation will require dedication and, at times, sacrifice. So, take comfort in knowing you will have this trusted framework to guide your decision making to maintain a stable, lucrative career.

Here are universal job expectations to direct you toward predictable, enjoyable, and rewarding work:

1. Be on time.
2. Be honest.
3. Be predictable.
4. Be prepared.
5. Speak professionally.
6. Accept feedback and learn from mistakes.
7. Seek opportunities to be helpful.

## 1. Be on time.

Being on time is the most straightforward and achievable of the seven guidelines. And it is one of the easiest displays of respect for others who count on you. However, many people routinely struggle with it. Failure to be on time is often a reflection of improper planning and not following a set routine. From the moment you wake up, your day can be compartmentalized into small, predictable tasks. You can incrementally map out your day prior to work with your pre-work activities. All it takes is a little planning.

We encourage you to take a few minutes every week to think about anything you want to accomplish prior to work and estimate the amount of time these tasks will take. This planning is crucial and will allow you to set aside the appropriate amount of time before work and adjust your sleep, activity, and departure times accordingly. Your routine can vary each day of the week, if needed, and when you anticipate and allot the appropriate amounts of time, you can adjust your pre-work schedule and still arrive for work as planned.

Routines are fundamental to dentistry, so get used to making one and following it. Dental procedures are often executed with the same steps in the same sequences, often taking predictable amounts of time. A little bit of buffer time may be added to an appointment to ensure completion of the visit prior to the next patient's appointment. This same concept should be applied to your routine prior to work. Add a few minutes to your calculations for pre-work activities so you can allow for minor setbacks and delays.

Most employers will expect you to arrive to work well before the first scheduled patient appointment time. Whatever time your employer sets as the start time of your workday, plan to be ten minutes early. Arriving slightly early shows your employer you have initiative, are predictable, and can be relied upon.

Use the ten-minutes-early start time as the benchmark for your planning. Backtrack from this time and add in your commute, breakfast—or any meal, depending on your work schedule—and all pre-work activities as part of your weekly planning. Add a little bit of buffer time between planned activities and commuting for unexpected delays. Then, you will have a start time for all pre-work activities and can set an alarm for when you need to wake up—or begin your pre-work activities—and when you must depart to arrive to work predictably. Now, go about your routine and adjust timing as necessary.

When did you arrive? Did you arrive much more than ten minutes early? Were you on time or slightly late? Do not worry, your employer will be somewhat flexible regarding your arrival time in the first few days of your new job as you get adjusted to commuting and traffic. However, beyond a day or two after your start date, you will be expected to be consistent. Tweak your departure time so you can predictably arrive early and stick to your timeline every workday.

With this new schedule, you will find your time before work is less stressful, and your employer will appreciate your consistency. Sickness and emergencies happen, so if you experience a significant setback for any reason, notify your employer as soon as you know you will not arrive as planned.

## 2. Be honest.

Honesty is fundamental to every aspect of healthcare. From working with coworkers, to patients, and all parties in between, honesty is critical in every interaction to maintain safety and confidence in clinical care. Many patients are unfamiliar with routine dental procedures and rely on the dental team to communicate truthfully about what may be experienced before, during, and after dental treatment. Accurately communicating with a patient about their anticipated dental experiences will build trust and, hopefully, loyalty to you and the dental practice. Honesty is a practiced behavior, and committing to this character trait takes routine dedication.

*Rule of thumb: Do not lie about anything.* Any time you are dishonest for any reason, you undermine the integrity of the work environment. Every step in a dental procedure is important, and many are performed without a dentist directly watching. The dentist and your coworkers will rely on you to perform your duties as trained to keep patients and staff safe. Cutting corners will often lead to more costly treatment and can jeopardize your health, as well as the patient's, and the practice's reputation. You do not have to always like your coworkers or your employer, but you must respect and trust them so patients can receive the safe care they deserve.

Many workplaces have a zero tolerance policy with dishonesty, even if the infraction seems miniscule or harmless. There is no place for deception in healthcare. As your comfort level builds in the workplace, you may be tempted to be dishonest in small ways. You may find redundancy in routinely checking equipment and performing mundane tasks and may wish to skip duties you feel are not necessary. You may also want additional time off work and contemplate calling in sick to get it. Choosing not to perform your job as expected and disregarding office protocols are forms of dishonesty. Even though these decisions may seem trivial, you will be putting additional strain on the dental team. Sickness will inevitably cause you to legitimately miss time from work, so just be honest. If you need to miss work, be truthful with the reason.

## 3. Be predictable.

In dental assisting and the workplace, predictability is highly valued and encouraged. It is critical to providing quality, consistent dentistry, no matter the day of the week, the patient in the chair, or any personal challenges you may be experiencing at home. Be predictable for the right reasons. A strong work ethic and positive attitude are expected once you walk into the office and for the rest of the workday. Strive for predictability in your *workflow, disposition*, and *behavior*.

Your workflow should be repeatable. Despite there being a wide range of clinical procedures performed in dental offices, it is important that similar procedures be executed with minimal variations. Consistency is key. So, follow the same procedural steps as trained unless instructed otherwise. We will cover standard dental procedures in more detail later.

Your disposition should be calm, collected, and courteous, no matter the patient's emotional state. The interactions between dentist and dental assistant should be calculated and seamless. With repetition, dental assistants should be able to anticipate the doctor's next moves and vice versa throughout an entire procedure.

Even when implementing the best techniques, dentistry can be challenging for all parties involved. From the first call a patient makes to the day a procedure is performed, many patients are apprehensive due to negative past experiences or hearing about other accounts of traumatic dental appointments from friends, family, or an online search. In order to provide quality dental care, patients must be directed and encouraged every step of the way. Sometimes patients just need the assurance they will get through a procedure, no matter how simple it may seem to you. Consistency and diligence will demonstrate you can be relied upon.

Often, your subtle behaviors with coworkers will impact how patients perceive the practice. Have a positive attitude with your colleagues. Dentistry can be emotionally taxing, and it may be easier to limit your emotional grace strictly to patients. But your team members will thrive when you extend compassion to everyone in the office. Many team members will just appreciate continued dependability and work ethic. If you become available during the workday, seek opportunities to assist other team members. Dental assistants who have predictable work ethics and attitudes are often highly valued and well-compensated.

## 4. Be prepared.

Presence of mind will allow you to calmly assist chairside, and your demeanor will reflect your understanding and planning prior to a patient's appointment. Every dental assistant is capable of being prepared if they take time to think through planned procedures and have the appropriate supplies and treatment room ready. This means a patient's appointment starts well before they arrive. A room must be prepared, and a dental assistant will need to think through every procedural step and set up accordingly.

Start with imagining a patient walking into the treatment room and sitting down. Do you have the patient's napkin, napkin chain, and safety glasses ready? Is the patient having a filling done today? Do you have the topical, anesthetic, and appropriate instruments and supplies? Have you tested the equipment to make sure the equipment is turned on and working? Imagine all the steps of an appointment and check the room to make sure you have what you need. You will find more information about basic dental supplies in the "Set-up and Fillings" section.

If you realize you are unfamiliar with a certain procedure, and you do not know what supplies are needed, communicate with your dentist or more experienced team members. Ideally, ask for clarification before the patient is seated in the treatment room. Having this discussion privately, preceding the appointment, will allow you to learn the intricacies of the upcoming procedure without unnecessarily extending the patient's appointment time and undermining your credibility with the patient. This level of anticipation is critical because if you do not understand the steps involved in the procedure, you will not be able to anticipate the workflow nor meet clinical expectations.

Take time to learn appointment workflow and how the dentist operates. Since many treatment steps are repetitive, make sure to learn the appropriate sequence of steps and commit them to memory. Dental assisting, like any profession, requires study and practice to become proficient. Mistakes may happen while you assist, so it is important to learn from these experiences and not consistently make the same mistakes in the future. **Helpful hint:** *Keep a small notepad and pen with you.* If you make an error during an appointment, make note of it so you can review and remember areas for improvement at the end of the day. Dental assisting is a fast-paced career that requires steadfast attention. Applying the level of focus required in patient care can easily derail your train of thought for other office duties. A notepad and pen will help you remember to return to certain tasks before the end of the day. New assistants will not be expected to know everything; however, the fundamentals explained in this book should be well-understood as you start your first dental assisting job.

## 5. Speak professionally.

At the heart of professionalism in dentistry is knowing your patients well enough to respect personal boundaries and maintain a calm environment for care. This guideline may be the most challenging to convey to a broad audience because respect is not communicated in a universal manner across all backgrounds, and expectations of conduct vary. Even patients within the same practice will have a wide variety of preferences and expectations. Some patients are more open and feel more comfortable when talking about themselves, while others are more guarded and prefer little conversation. You must navigate some level of uncertainty during your initial interactions with patients as you learn their dispositions and preferences.

Here are some guidelines for patient interactions:

- Keep your language appropriate and conversation light. Allow patients to direct any initial conversations so you can gauge personalities and what topics put patients at ease. Some patients may use profanity jokingly or as a result of being anxious or in pain. Whether profanity is used in jest, due to physical discomfort, or unclearly provoked, respond unanimously with assurance to the patient that the dental team will give full attention to their needs. Often, communicating sincerely with patients redirects conversations professionally.

- Do not use profanity even if a patient does. Make sure your language reflects the expectations of the office. You must understand workplace culture and what your employer expects in your daily behavior. In most private practice offices, the dentist will set expectations and will establish and direct the office's mission or purpose.
- Look to the dentist for leadership and observe how different job roles in the office work together. How do team members communicate and work together? Are there clear expectations to follow? Do not hesitate to ask for clarification if you need it.
- How does the dentist like to be addressed by the team and in front of patients? When in doubt, address dentists with the professional title of "Doctor" unless you are told otherwise. The same goes for addressing patients who are also doctors, even if they are retired.

Your success with patient interactions and maintaining professionalism depends on your ability to listen, be personable, and communicate well. If you are new to a work team, ask other individuals at your office about the patients you will see so you can learn about their dispositions and histories with the practice. If a patient interaction does not go as smoothly as you wished, ask for feedback and pointers from your teammates.

If you ever experience inappropriate or unwanted interactions from anyone at the office, including patients, your dentist should be notified immediately. It is the dentist's responsibility to ensure the health, safety, and well-being of all clinical team members. If you feel any concerns about your health and safety are not adequately addressed, you can contact the Occupational Safety and Health Administration (OSHA) at www.osha.gov and find additional resources.

## 6. Accept feedback and learn from mistakes.

One of the most challenging aspects of professional growth is accepting constructive criticism. When your employer brings up techniques or behaviors in need of modification, it can be easy to respond emotionally and totally disregard the content of the message. Rather than allowing emotions to drive these conversations, listen to feedback and ask for clarification so you can better understand the presented concerns. **Helpful hint:** *Do not allow your emotions to distract you from learning and improving.* If you feel offended by any feedback, allow volatile emotions to subside before responding so you can respond appropriately and objectively.

Another challenge is implementing newly modified techniques once feedback has been received. Many people take comfort in routine and performing tasks certain ways. This reality can lead to complacency and resistance to change. Often, changing the way a task is performed can, at first, make a procedure feel more challenging than it was originally. **Helpful hint:** *Be patient and apply new methods consistently.* With time, the modifications will feel more natural.

The truth is dentistry is a constantly evolving profession. As you read this, new technologies are emerging to make dental procedures more efficient and less daunting for patients. Our techniques for providing dental care must also evolve with time. Even how we interact with patients will adapt and change as new communication platforms make other ways of engaging with patients obsolete. Staying relevant and accessible is critical for a small business to survive and prosper.

Change is inevitable. So, strive to take feedback with an open mind. It is simply part of your professional journey. Every aspect of your clinical care will transform with experience. As you implement modified techniques, ask if your new methods are meeting expectations. **Helpful hint:** *Asking for confirmation shows team members you understood constructive feedback and are committed to making necessary improvements.*

## 7. Seek opportunities to be helpful.

When you start a new job, you may be presented with a job description outlining specific duties. Maybe your employer will tell you certain tasks must be completed each day. If there is uncertainty in your job description, make sure to speak with your employer to clarify daily expectations. This information is an excellent resource for how to prioritize your time in accordance to your specific office duties.

As you address your specific office responsibilities, you may find you have some spare time in between tasks. If so, seek other ways to be helpful. Some assistants may have limited success in dentistry if they view their job duties as the only tasks they must complete to be successful employees. When focusing solely on your specific duties, you may fail to see the bigger picture of why you were hired.

How can you add value to the practice?

- Remember your purpose. You were hired to allow a business to function more effectively. It can be easy to have tunnel vision and focus only on a list of tasks instead of being helpful to others and striving to be a team asset.
- Team members quickly recognize unfair work burdens. If you have addressed your office duties and are available, you should offer your assistance and alleviate stress and frustration of team members who are managing more challenging or time-intensive work duties.
- In a dental office, no task is of greater importance than caring for patients in a personal and professional manner. If you are available, check on patients who may be waiting to be seen by the dentist. This thoughtful attention to patients builds rapport and makes patients feel cared for. Even brief conversations can calm patients who may be becoming anxious or impatient.

You are soon to be an integral part of a business, and you must be aware of the other job roles at the dental office. If you can meet your job expectations while also helping your team members successfully execute their respective roles, you will be helping the overall business thrive. Making use of any spare time to help provide excellent patient experiences and assist coworkers on tasks allows business operations to flow more smoothly and efficiently. Your work ethic will be recognized, and your team will greatly value your support.

As you apply yourself in helpful ways, be mindful of the following:

- Ask for additional training and expand your responsibilities if you are available after completing your daily duties. Helping the business function more effectively will, in turn, warrant growth in your compensation and provide you with job security.
- Dental equipment is expensive and must be handled carefully and with proper training. If you are unfamiliar with a new task, make sure you receive proper instruction and communicate with the dentist and your coworkers as you plan to take on new tasks.

These seven guidelines form a code of conduct that will ensure your success. Each guiding principle will benefit you in unique ways if you regularly commit to them. With any code of conduct, your personal accountability will determine if it holds lasting value for you. If you dedicate yourself to the seven guidelines, you are guaranteed to navigate your workdays with less stress, knowing you always have a blueprint to guide your decision making.

Reinforce your learning by listing the seven guidelines for success here:

1.
2.
3.
4.
5.
6.
7.

The content of this book moving forward will shift from how to professionally interact with others to habits and behaviors to aid in clinical success in chairside dental assisting. There are countless clinical skills necessary to be an excellent dental assistant. You must pair your reading and study with hands-on experiences, and the best way to reinforce your knowledge is in a clinical setting. As you become more comfortable and confident as a dental assistant, continue to search for new ways to improve your chairside skills. The best dental assistants are always looking to improve and never stop learning.

# The Office

Welcome to your new workplace! Below is a picture of a typical dental *operatory*. An operatory is a treatment room where dental procedures are performed. Every dental office is different, but you will find that most are equipped with similar instruments for dentistry.

*Image 1*

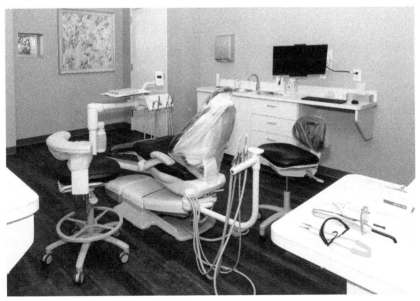

In the center of Image 1, you can see a patient chair with a plastic barrier, as well as equipment to the right and behind the chair, covered with plastic. Plastic barriers are commonly used to reduce contamination to equipment and allow ease of cleaning.

## Room turnover

When a patient walks into the operatory, all working surfaces and equipment must be safe for use. There are different standards of cleaning, or *infection control*, for surfaces patients touch versus instruments used within the mouth. Surfaces fixed in a room, like chairs and countertops, must be wiped with disinfectants when contaminated. Instruments that have direct contact with teeth and tissues must be sterilized. It is important to distinguish the difference between disinfection and sterilization.

*Disinfection* is the reduction of infectious material from surfaces that may have been contaminated with blood, saliva, bacteria, and viruses. Disinfectants render the surfaces non-infectious—i.e., the contaminants are reduced to such small levels, diseases are very unlikely to be transmitted from the affected surfaces. Disinfection does not mean bacteria or viruses are totally eliminated from the surfaces after disinfectant use. There are still small traces of microorganisms, just not enough to transmit disease. Disinfectants do not make surfaces sterile. Common brands of disinfectants advertise being effective at killing a very high percentage of germs, so it can be assumed that a very low percentage of germs will remain on the surface.

*Sterilization* is a process that eliminates all microorganisms. Sterilization is critical for instruments used in the mouth. There are many different methods of sterilization, but the most common method uses a machine called an *autoclave*. An autoclave uses high temperatures, steam, and pressure to eliminate all traces of microorganisms on instruments. Instruments must be heat-resistant at high temperatures to be sterilized in an autoclave, or they will melt and be destroyed.

Before instruments enter an autoclave, they must be wiped down and soaked in an *ultrasonic bath*. The ultrasonic bath removes debris with vibration and liquid enzymes before instruments are sterilized. After the ultrasonic, cassettes are wrapped in sterilization paper and loose instruments are placed in sterilization pouches prior to being placed in the autoclave for sterilization. Approved wrapping paper and sealable pouches allow instruments to be sterilized and stored for later use. Often, these materials will have an indicator pattern that changes in the autoclave, signaling these materials have been successfully sterilized.

Even if a room looks clean, it may not be. Contamination can be microscopic and unseen by the naked eye. So, make sure to clearly communicate with team members if there is any doubt a room may be clean prior to use. If an instrument is dropped, it must be treated as soiled even if no visible debris is present. **Important note:** *Never use a dropped instrument on a patient.* Microorganisms cover the floor and can be harmful if introduced to the mouth. If an instrument is dropped mid-treatment, seek direction from the dentist if you need to clean or replace the instrument immediately.

## How do you clean a room?

One of your job duties will be to clean and prepare rooms between appointments, restoring a room to order (refer to Image 1). This task is often referred to as room turnover. Once a procedure is performed, and a patient is dismissed, you will need to dispose of single-use materials, take instruments to the sterilization station, and clean working surfaces. Here are steps to follow:

1. Organize all the contaminated materials. All cotton products— cotton rolls, gauze, dry angles, cotton pellets, patient napkin, etc.—single-use plastic brushes, and plastic suction tips used during treatment are disposable and must be thrown away after use. Gather all disposables and place them in the plastic barrier from the head of the chair, turning it into a trash bag. Now you will be left with only reusable materials, which need to be wiped, sterilized, or both.

2. Organize and inspect the cassette. A *cassette*, shown in Image 2, is a container for organizing and transporting instruments. The

type of container, or cassette, will vary between practices. Some are durable plastic, and others are metal. The lid of the cassette in the image below is not shown, which allows the cassette to be closed for transport.

*Image 2*

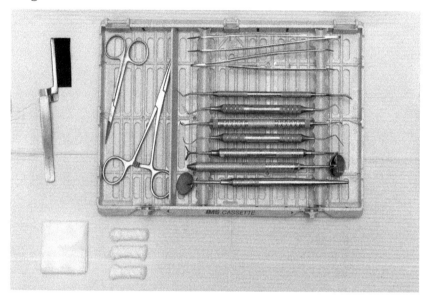

3. Inspect instruments for damage and debris. If there is any visible debris present on the instruments, it needs to be wiped away prior to closing the cassette. Any bulk debris or blood left on instruments may not be effectively removed in the ultrasonic bath, and remnants will strongly adhere to instruments in the autoclave. Taking a moment to wipe the debris off the instruments prior to sterilization will keep them in pristine condition and will save you time and energy trying to remove unsightly deposits after instruments are autoclaved.

4. Make sure all the instruments are lined up properly and close the cassette for transport. If instruments are placed too close to the edge, they can be easily broken by closing the lid, which is a

costly mistake. If any instrument appears broken, bring it to the attention of the dentist.

5. Once trash has been collected, and the cassette is organized, you can take the cassette to the sterilization station and return to the operatory for final cleaning steps. **Helpful hint:** *If the material is made of cotton, it is disposable.* If the material is not made of cotton, ask the dentist if it is disposable before throwing it away.

6. Spray and wipe all working surfaces: chairs, suction and handpiece tubing, countertops, and any other surfaces touched with contaminated, gloved hands. All that should remain in the room now should be the mounted equipment, with no trash present. Wipe all surfaces with disinfectant and inspect for any visible debris.

   - *Spray-wipe-spray*: Each office may have preferred disinfectants and steps for cleaning surfaces. Often, the spray-wipe-spray method is taught and expected. This method involves spraying surfaces with disinfectant, wiping surfaces, spraying the surfaces again with disinfectant, and leaving surfaces to dry. This is an effective method of disinfection.

7. Check and clear the floor for any materials, instruments, or disposables that may have fallen during treatment.

8. Set up the room for the next patient.

# Set-up and Filling Terminology

Once you know how to thoroughly clean a room and restore it to the status shown in Image 1 on page 25, you need to know how to set up for a filling appointment. *Fillings* are one of the most common procedures performed in dental offices. Fillings, or resins, refer to a type of dental restoration involving the removal and reconstruction of damaged tooth structure. A simplified overview of a basic filling appointment goes as follows:

1. A patient is seated in an operatory and provided proper safety gear. Often, patients will be required to wear safety glasses to protect the eyes from aerosol debris, water spray, and instruments. Removal of tooth decay generates dust and aerosol particles, which necessitates protective eyewear for patients and clinical staff.

2. The dentist enters the room and anesthetizes the patient. Prior to delivering a dental injection, topical gel will be placed on the cheek by the planned injection site. It provides a brief numbing sensation, which minimizes discomfort for the duration of a dental injection. The dental injection, or shot, provides profound local anesthesia so the dental procedure is not painful to the patient. Local anesthesia allows the numbness to be isolated

to the mouth so patients can be conscious during dental treatment.

3. The dentist removes any broken or decayed tooth structure with a dental drill, using copious amounts of water, while the dental assistant applies suction and retracts the lip, cheek, and tongue.

4. When the appropriate adjustments are made, the affected tooth can be repaired. The tooth structure is made ready by first applying an *etchant* and thoroughly rinsing with water and air-drying. The etchant, or "etch," creates microscopic texture on the tooth, which allows dental materials to attach and bond to the tooth. Enamel that is etched and dried will have a lighter, chalkier appearance.

5. Then a desensitizer is applied to the tooth and dried. The inner layers of teeth are very sensitive and dental desensitizers help clean the prepared surface and prevent lasting sensitivity after teeth are repaired.

6. After the desensitizer is dried, primer and bonding agents are applied to the tooth. Very small brushes are used to paint solutions on the tooth structure. The bonding agents integrate with the texture created by the etch. The bonding agents must be thinned on the tooth, which involves applying five seconds of continuous air spray, or using small brushes to remove excess. A curing light is used to affix the bonding agent to the tooth.

7. Once the tooth has primer and bonding agent applied, a restorative material can be placed on the tooth and cured. Many restorative, or filling, materials are soft when they are applied to the tooth and the *curing light* hardens them. After the filling is cured, all that remains is making small adjustments with dental drills so the filling fits appropriately with the patient's bite and is smooth.

In order to set up and assist in filling procedures, you will need to be familiar with basic dental terminology:

- **Anesthetic:** solution stored in glass carpules (cartridges) and extruded through a syringe (needle)
- **Articulating paper:** thin, colored paper (often blue) a patient bites on to check their occlusion (bite) after a filling
- **Bur:** dental drill bit; a small, metal, removable bit which rotates in the drill and can cut tooth structure
- **Cavity:** a hole in a tooth
- **Cure/curing:** a process that transitions a material to its desired state through polymerization and; transitions the material from a soft, moveable consistency to a hard, durable consistency
- **Curing light:** a handheld device that emits blue light to cure, polymerize, or harden filling materials; performed in timed sessions, often five to twenty seconds
- **Dappen dish:** container made of glass or plastic to hold a few drops of solution (desensitizer, primer, or bonding agents)
- **Decay:** tooth structure compromised by acid-producing bacteria; also known as *caries* a microbial process rendering tooth structure soft and structurally vulnerable; dentists often check for decay with an explorer
- **Dentin:** middle layer of a tooth
- **Desensitizer:** liquid applied with a brush directly after the tooth is etched and dried; helps clean the preparation and reduce tooth sensitivity following a filling procedure
- **Enamel:** outer layer of a tooth
- **Etch:** gel (often blue) placed on teeth after decay is removed; first step after decay is removed to prepare a tooth for a filling
- **Explorer:** a fine-tipped instrument used for checking teeth and restorations; if the explorer penetrates the tooth structure and "sticks," there is a cavity
- **Filling:** doughy (or more fluid) material used to rebuild broken or decayed teeth; white, tooth-colored fillings require a blue light so the material can be cured

- **Handpiece:** a dental drill used to remove decay, broken tooth structure, and adjust restorations; uses water spray to protect teeth while repairs are made
- **Matrix:** a clear or metal band used to assist in filling placement; can be secured around prepared teeth and allow for teeth to be rebuilt
- **Preparation:** affected tooth surfaces after decay or broken structure is removed prior to restoration
- **Prime and Bond:** liquid applied with a brush before the filling material is placed, the liquid is air-thinned for five seconds and then cured for ten seconds
- **Pulp:** inner layer of a tooth with blood vessels and nerves
- **Shade:** specific color of a filling material; shades are on a gradient classified by letters and numbers so material selection can be precise (e.g., A2, B1, C3, D4, etc.)
- **Shade Guide:** a tool used to select the proper shade for a restoration
- **Topical:** numbing gel placed on tissue prior to an injection
- **Wedge:** a triangular piece of wood or plastic used to apply pressure against a matrix and a tooth during filling placement; pressure allows materials to be placed without leaking

*Image 3: Closed cassette*

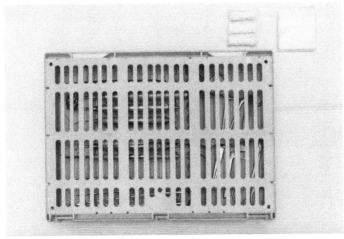

*Image 4: Bur block, highspeed handpiece (red stripe), slow speed handpiece (blue stripe), and corresponding burs*

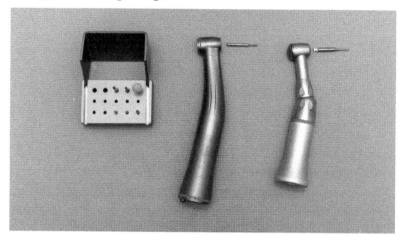

*Image 5: Articulating paper, 2x2 gauze, cotton rolls, cassette, air/water syringe, handpieces, and burs set up*

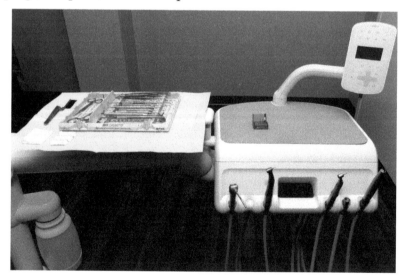

After learning the sequence of a filling appointment and the respective dental materials, it is important to know descriptive terminology for tooth surfaces. Teeth have anatomic landmarks, so when you look at a tooth, it is helpful to think in terms of cardinal directions. Traditionally, cardinal directions refer to those on a compass, allowing you to think spatially in regards to locations on a map. A compass allows you to navigate between locations and communicate where one destination is in relationship to another.

The ability to identify and navigate between distinct regions is also important when evaluating and treating teeth. The dentist and dental assistant must communicate where teeth need attention, so dental materials, suction, air, water, and curing light can be delivered with precision and accuracy in the mouth. Recognizing and using appropriate terminology will expedite appointments with a common understanding of treatment objectives and the technical skills that follow.

The main anatomic cardinal directions for teeth are *incisal* and *occlusal*; *gingival, facial,* and *buccal*; *lingual, mesial,* and *distal*. Incisal and occlusal refer to the biting edge of the tooth. Gingival refers to the section of the tooth closest to the gums or gingiva. Facial or buccal refers to the side of the tooth that faces the lip or cheek. Lingual refers to the side of the tooth that faces the tongue. Mesial refers to the side of the tooth that is positioned to the patient's midline or center of the patient's lips. Distal refers to the side of the tooth that faces the back of the patient's mouth.

Between the four main cardinal directions, north, south, east, and west are intercardinal directions, which are northeast, northwest, southeast, and southwest. These are even more specific terms describing the regions in between cardinal directions. Similarly in dentistry, terminology can be further specified to distinguish more narrow anatomic regions.

Directional, anatomic terms may be combined with the letter "o," to create variations like *mesiofacial, distolingual, incisofacial,* etc. These terms identify regions of the tooth that are near line angles where regions merge. For example, if a dentist asks you to cure the mesiolingual of a tooth, you will be expected to place the curing light on the tongue side of the tooth, toward the patient's midline. In contrast, if the dentist directs you to cure the distolingual, you will be expected to place the curing light on the tongue side of the tooth more toward the back of the mouth.

As you can imagine, there are many ways to combine these terms to increase precision. As long as you understand the main anatomic cardinal directions, you will be able to decipher combinations that describe distinct regions of teeth during procedures. These variations of dental terminology will significantly broaden your dental vocabulary, and subsequently, your ability to understand clinical instructions and execute clinical responsibilities.

The terms *anterior* and *posterior* are more general anatomical terms. In dentistry, anterior refers to the region closer to the front of the mouth and posterior refers to the region closer to the back of the mouth. These more general terms are often used to direct the positioning of the suction, where the instrument has a wider field of effective use. In essence, you can position the suction in many different regions during treatment and still provide adequate suction. Do not hesitate to ask for confirmation that you are in an acceptable position, especially for curing restorations. The curing light has a narrow field of effective use, and slight errors in positioning may prevent the restoration from being properly cured.

Now that you know the workflow and necessary terminology, you will be able to respond appropriately during clinical procedures, anticipate procedural steps, and communicate professionally chairside. As you recognize typical workflow, be ready to present the corresponding materials and instruments to the dentist. It is important to have these items in hand and ready for exchange, even before the dentist asks. It is better to display anticipation and present materials even if you are not certain they are needed rather than wait empty-handed for instruction.

To summarize:
- **Incisal/occlusal:** biting edge of tooth
- **Gingival:** surface by gumline
- **Facial/buccal:** cheek side of tooth
- **Lingual:** surface by tongue
- **Mesial:** side of tooth closest to midline
- **Distal:** side of tooth closest to back of mouth
- **Anterior:** region toward front of mouth
- **Posterior:** region toward back of mouth

## Filling Procedure and Necessary Materials

| Steps | Materials |
|---|---|
| Seat patient | Safety glasses and napkin |
| Anesthetize | Topical and anesthetic in syringe |
| Prepare tooth | Handpiece(s) with burs<br>Cassette<br>Cotton rolls and tools for isolation<br>2x2 gauze |
| Prepare to restore | Matrix and wedge<br>  (if multiple surface filling)<br>Etch<br>Desensitizer<br>Prime and bond<br>Microbrushes<br>Dappen dish |
| Cure | Curing light |
| Check occlusion | Articulating paper<br>Polishing burs<br>Sanding strips (if multiple surface filling) |
| Check contacts | Floss |

*Image 6*

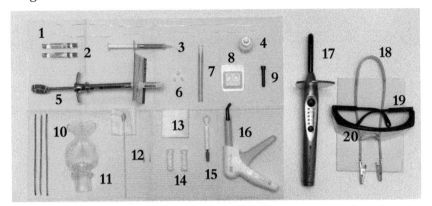

Name the common materials for filling appointment found in the image above:

1.
2.
3.
4.
5.
6.
7.
8.
9.
10.
11.
12.
13.
14.
15.
16.
17.
18.
19.
20.

*Key can be found at the end of the book.

# Common Dental Procedures

There are three common factors that greatly influence restorative dentistry needs for patients: improper hygiene, dental trauma, and patient biology. The repercussions of improper hygiene most frequently pose the need for dental treatment. Bacteria live in the mouth and survive by eating foods humans eat. When a person consumes a meal, bacteria also consume the food. Bacteria produce acids as they digest, and these acid byproducts damage teeth. If teeth are not properly cleaned after meals, food remnants are left in the mouth longer, allowing bacteria to feast longer, and as a result, more damaging acids harm the tooth structure. This bacterial damage can lead to tooth destruction, infection, and possibly complex dental treatments.

To better understand the risks bacterial damage poses to tooth structure, it is important to review the anatomy of a tooth. The consistency of the tooth structure is very similar to bones in the human body. The strong outer layer of a tooth is called *enamel*, which protects the inner layers of the tooth and allows patients to function. At the center of teeth are nerves and blood vessels that allow our teeth to sense temperatures and pressures. Between the strong outer layer of the tooth and the soft innermost layer of a tooth housing the vasculature and innervation, there is a middle layer called *dentin*. Dentin is a yellow, softer layer compared to enamel and has some moderate strength and durability.

Any time the outer layer of the teeth is damaged, patients are at risk of experiencing pain, discomfort, or dysfunction in their mouths.

Routine brushing and flossing remove debris from the mouth and minimize the harmful effects of bacteria. Patient diet also impacts how easily bacteria survive in the oral cavity. Foods high in sugars and carbohydrates are more readily digested by bacteria and allow bacteria to quickly produce detrimental acids. Diets comprised of whole foods, low in sugar, tend to have a lower risk of promoting tooth decay, as these foods are more challenging for bacteria to digest. Even if a patient observes a healthy diet, poor oral hygiene can still allow bacterial acids to slowly damage tooth structure, causing a wide array of dental maladies.

Healthy diets and excellent hygiene will not completely eradicate the need for restorative dental procedures. Sometimes, patients with healthy teeth encounter dental trauma. For example, a patient could experience a car crash where the force of the collision imposes dental injuries. Sports injuries commonly cause trauma that warrants dental treatment. Patients may clench and grind their teeth due to psychological conditions or as a side effect of medication, which can damage otherwise healthy teeth. Any strong forces applied to teeth can cause chips or fractures. Under extreme forces, teeth and surrounding structures can break significantly, leading to multidisciplinary dental care.

Dentistry can also serve to restore esthetics for patients with biologic tooth abnormalities. Teeth develop in the womb and throughout childhood and adolescence. Sometimes, due to genetic or environmental factors, teeth develop abnormally or fail to develop at all. There are countless health conditions that can affect tooth structure. Occasionally, teeth can be missing or structurally compromised to the point where dental work is necessary to help patients function and interact in society. Teeth are visible in face-to-face interactions, and if obvious asymmetries and structural abnormalities are present, unpleasant assumptions may be made about the character of an individual who has irregular or missing teeth. Esthetic dentistry can allow patients to interact with confidence, without concern that their teeth will be a distraction.

These are the main causes for dental treatments, but there are countless others that can cause patients to need and desire dental treatment. Doctors are not yet able to regrow damaged permanent teeth, so dentists have learned and developed techniques to address many dental problems. Here are the descriptions of some of the most common dental procedures:

- **Crown:** Crowns restore the appearance and function of natural teeth. If a tooth is significantly damaged, and a filling will not adequately repair the tooth, a crown may be needed. Crowns, often referred to as *caps*, are made of strong porcelain or metal and cover the whole outer surface of a tooth. In order to provide a crown for a patient, a tooth is often reduced in size with a bur, and an impression is taken. Once a crown is made, either by a dental lab or with in-office equipment, it can be cemented to the tooth.

- **Extraction:** Extraction is the process of removing a tooth. If a tooth is broken beyond repair, or if the patient does not wish to have restorative treatment provided, removing a tooth could be the best option for a patient. Sometimes to effectively straighten teeth with orthodontics, a poorly positioned tooth may need to be removed. In order to remove the tooth, pressure is placed around the supporting periodontal ligaments, allowing the tooth to be elevated and taken out of the mouth. After an extraction, the *socket*, or space where a tooth once resided, is cleaned.

- **Impression:** An impression is a digital or physical record of a patient's mouth, which can allow for teeth to be evaluated. Physical impressions involve mixing a putty material and placing it over the teeth. Once the material sets (cures), after a specific set time, it can be removed from the patient's mouth, rendering a negative duplication of the patient's teeth. Dental models can be made from placing stone mix into the impression, creating an accurate stone representation of a patient's teeth, which can be used to educate patients or build a dental prosthesis. Digital impressions are taken from a scanner, a device that takes a series of pictures of a patient's teeth, forming an accurate three-dimensional, digital model.

- **Root Canal:** Root canals refer to the procedure of removing and cleaning the nerve, *pulp*, chamber within a tooth and placing a root canal filling. Sometimes, cavities extend so deeply within the tooth, the blood vessels and nerves become infected. It is also possible that a tooth experiences trauma that disturbs the pulp and causes irreversible damage. In these scenarios, the compromised nerve fibers and blood vessels can be removed from the tooth, and a filling within the root is placed.

# Ergonomics and Suction

*E*rgonomics refers to how your body is positioned to reduce physical stress. Good posture and proper hand control and positioning will reduce the risk of physical injury when dental assisting. Poor posture will not likely have immediate negative consequences; however, over time, the physical strain of poor posture can result in injuries to your muscles, joints, and nervous system. Using proper form and techniques will prevent unnecessary work-related stress on your body, but it will not completely prevent all muscle and joint stress.

It is important to maintain your physical health and core strength so you can meet the physical demands of dental assisting over a long career. Core strength will give your back proper support as you move. Neck and back injuries are common for dentists and assistants, so protect yourself with routine stretching and exercise. Wearing comfortable, closed-toed shoes will allow you to move and stand for longer periods with good posture and will protect your feet if materials are dropped.

In order to preserve your back and neck muscles from unwarranted strain, position yourself close to the patient. You do not want to hunch or lean over the patient. If the dentist operates on the right side of the patient, then position yourself by the patient's left shoulder so you can look down the bridge of your nose to the patient without straining your neck. Your view of the patient must be at a higher vantage point than the dentist's.

Many assistants are more comfortable standing next to the patient, which often achieves the appropriate view. Standing is encouraged as the default assisting position. The higher vantage point compared to the dentist is important; you can have quick access and view of dental materials while also monitoring the patient and providing suction. Standing will also ensure you are not leaning from the arm of a chair in poor posture. Keep your feet shoulder-width apart and planted, with your back straight. Once you are in a good position, you will be able to provide better suction and isolation during the dental procedure. Appropriate suction and isolation are the most important clinical aspects of chairside assisting.

There are multiple instruments you will need easily accessible to affectively maintain the working field for the dentist. Your most common instrument for retraction, isolation, and suction will be the *high-volume suction*, or HVAC. Many new assistants are hesitant to use the HVAC because it is larger and requires more control and coordination. The tubing is also thicker, which requires assertive use and controlled manipulation. But no other device removes the same volume of debris, water, and saliva as the HVAC, so become familiar with and confident in using it.

*Image 7*

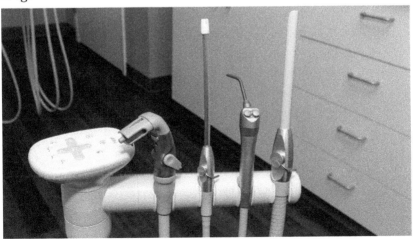

Image 7 shows some typical instruments that will be accessible for a dental assistant. From left to right, you see the bite block suction, low volume suction, air-water syringe, and the HVAC. In the image, the HVAC has a pink plastic suction tip.

*Image 8: Tangled tubing vs proper arrangement*

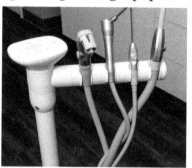 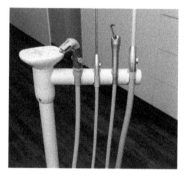

Observe how the image on the right has straight and organized tubing, whereas the tubing on the left is wrapped and tangled. Make sure the tubing stays untangled. Tangled equipment restricts movement and effective use and increases the risk of equipment becoming dislodged and falling to the floor unintentionally. Check the tubing for tangles throughout treatment and reorganize as necessary.

## High-volume handling

You can easily cause harm to the patient by not wielding the HVAC properly. Hold the suction from the metal connection base, where the disposable suction tip is inserted. Make sure not to secure your grip on the suction tip itself because it is removeable and can easily be dislodged, causing you to lose control of the suction and potentially injure the patient. Place the metal juncture in your hand like a pen. Now, use your pointer and middle finger to secure the suction. The proper grip is termed *modified pen grasp*.

*Image 9*

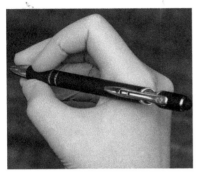
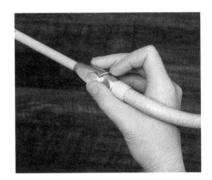

In the above right image, observe how the metal juncture between the disposable tip and the flexible tubing is safely in the hand. The pointer and middle finger are secure, with the on-and-off valve switch in contact with the pointer finger. This technique allows you to easily turn the suction on and off without changing its positioning or loosening your grip on the HVAC. You can easily practice the modified pen grasp with both hands and a writing instrument at home, as you will need to be comfortable managing the suction in either hand, depending on the clinical procedure.

Be very mindful that the disposable HVAC tip is hard plastic. The suction tip will be used to guide tissues out of the working field. Do not rest the plastic tip on the patient's gum tissue, even if said patient is numb. Pressing the plastic tip into gum tissues will cause trauma and possible ulcerations, which can make recovery from a dental procedure very painful once anesthetic wears off. If you need to steady your HVAC suction tip, use a cotton roll. A cotton roll can be placed in the patient's *vestibule*, the space between the lip and the gums, and pressures can be applied to the cotton roll with the HVAC tip without causing trauma.

# Radiography and Photography

One of your primary responsibilities as a dental assistant is taking dental X-rays. It is becoming increasingly common in dentistry to use digital photography in conjunction with radiography to educate patients and establish thorough records. Photography uses the reflection of light to capture images. With photography, there is often a flash, and the camera can interpret the volume of light and produce a picture. With X-ray technology, your handheld or mounted X-ray tube can be pointed at a sensor, and this equipment can send X-rays through an object to a sensor and produce a contrasted image of the object. Photos capture the outer surfaces of teeth. X-rays show you the internal aspects of teeth.

General concepts of radiography and photography will be covered in this section. You must have hands-on training to learn how to operate imaging technologies, but the general principles of radiography and photography are the same:

1. Position the patient.
2. Position your equipment, including lead apron when needed.
3. Instruct the patient to be still.
4. Take the image.
5. Evaluate your image for possible retake.

The quality of your image will be impacted by how well you execute the aforementioned steps. As you evaluate your X-rays and photos, think of each step. If your image is not ideal, try to identify which step infringed on your success and adjust your technique accordingly. One way to increase the likelihood of capturing a quality image is to educate the patient about the procedure and inform them how they can help you achieve success when images are taken.

Sometimes, technology malfunctions. However, this tends to be very rare. It is much more likely for technology to be used improperly, leading to poor images. The most common errors involve poor positioning; either the provider used an improper technique or had the patient (or sensor) in an improper position.

If you take an X-ray or a photograph and the image produced does not show the teeth you wanted to capture, but you see teeth in the image, you have a positioning error. You must adjust your position, the patient's position, or the position of your sensor before making another attempt. If you take an X-ray or photograph and no image is displayed at all, you may be experiencing a rare technological error and must notify your employer.

# The Next Steps

The journey to becoming a great dental assistant presents many unique challenges, new skills to learn and master, and rewards few individuals experience in their careers. Hopefully this information has served to broaden your understanding of dentistry, provided useful knowledge you can apply to your next job, and inspired you to develop clinical skills to excel as a dental assistant. Please use this information as an introductory guide and reference as you navigate your first steps in dental assisting. It is an exciting career, with each day presenting new and unique challenges, and we believe you can face each one with confidence should you apply proven behaviors to succeed in the workplace.

As you embark on the next steps of your career, remember every job is personal. Whether you choose to chairside assist or investigate another career path, how you treat and interact with other people will largely impact your professional success. Quality, professional relationships can add value to challenging work and sustain an environment where you can continuously learn and grow. How you treat people is just as important as providing excellent clinical service. Remember to learn, apply your knowledge, and improve every day.

You are now ready for the clinical training to develop hands-on dental assisting skills. As you navigate the next steps of your training and clinical practice, be confident. You have learned foundational concepts that will give your clinical skills purpose. Your clinical competency will flourish as you strive to meet the essential dentistry objectives you have thoroughly reviewed. Success will follow. We are so thankful you have taken the first steps in your dental assisting journey with us. The rest is up to you. You will be great!

Key to Image 3:

1. Floss
2. Anesthetic carpules
3. Etch/etchant (blue)
4. Desensitizer
5. Syringe
6. Cotton pellets
7. Microbrushes
8. Dappen dish
9. Prime and bond
10. Interproximal strips (sanding)
11. Bite block
12. Topical anesthetic (on cotton-tipped applicator)
13. 2 x 2 gauze
14. Cotton rolls
15. Matrix band
16. Composite gun (hand dispenser)
17. Curing light
18. Napkin chain
19. Napkin
20. Patient safety glasses

# Q & A with the Author,
# Robert E. Porter, DDS

1. What inspired you to write this book for dental assistants?

   *Early in my career as a dentist, I helped expand a team of dental assistants, and I quickly realized there are so many energetic and enthusiastic dental assistants entering the workforce with limited exposure to the breadth of responsibilities and work expectations in dentistry. The transition from dental assisting school to clinical practice is challenging as new assistants learn job expectations while trying to execute new skills. Often, I saw new dental assistants face similar struggles that could have been prevented with a little guidance and preparation. I felt a professional obligation to design a resource that could further educate, guide, and support dental assistants as they begin their careers. What if there were a guidebook that could make professional success predictable and easily attainable? The content of this book intertwines core values of the dental assisting profession with fundamental concepts of dentistry so that dental assistants can embark on new careers with confidence.*

2. How do you believe your book will impact the training of new dental assistants?

   *This book advocates for new dental assistants by providing clear objectives and explanations for common dental office procedures, and how specific behaviors and work habits can inspire professional growth. Many dental assistants aspire to enter the workforce and build careers that are financially and emotionally fulfilling. This book is designed to guide dental assistants through social and clinical scenarios so they are equipped for the diverse challenges involved with dental care and can achieve the careers they desire.*

*Dental assisting training will become more meaningful. Learning new skills and concepts is strengthened by visualizing information in different formats with explanations from various perspectives. This book diversifies understanding by providing descriptions of procedures, and why communication, technique, and consistency are important to dental care. This book serves as a helpful resource for dental assistants to add breadth to their understanding.*

3. Tell me about the importance of mentorship and continuous learning in the field of dentistry.

*Learning new skills can be mentally and physically challenging. It can be overwhelming to start from scratch, build expertise, and implement techniques of a skilled practitioner. Fortunately, not all lessons must be hard learned through the headaches of trial and error. Shared experiences can allow assistants to learn second-hand how to navigate a wide variety of scenarios. Sometimes this mentorship can be provided through personal connections, learning from more experienced individuals in your network. Alternatively, written and video resources can provide guidance to wider audiences.*

*Dental assistants can benefit from these various forms of mentorship, allowing them to effectively bypass many of the tribulations of learned experiences and apply proven methods for success. Often, experienced providers are willing to invest time to teach and coach newcomers, but the key is identifying those with experience and making the effort to connect and ask for help.*

*Not everyone has access to individuals who can provide quality mentorship, which presents the challenge of accessing clear, concise, and trusted information. This resource was designed to serve as a pocket mentor, a trusted resource that provides clear, need-to-know concepts to accelerate professional success. As your perspective and skills develop, continue the pursuit of more comprehensive information. Your personal knowledge will determine the quality of your clinical decisions, so continue to expand your understanding as you diversify your skills.*

4. What advice do you have for new dental assistants entering the field?
   *Ask questions. You will be surprised by what people teach you, and you will be even more surprised by how people treat you differently when they realize you want to learn.*

5. What do you hope dental assistants will take away from your book?
   *I hope dental assistants take comfort in knowing successful work habits, fundamental principles of dentistry, and the purpose of dental assisting duties. I believe if you develop an understanding of why certain techniques are important, you can better craft your professional skills in a way that is tailored to shared goals of the dental team. Ultimately, I want dental assistants to feel value, purpose, and the gratification that comes with meaningful careers.*

6. How do you think being a dentist writing a book for dental assistants offers a unique perspective as opposed to a dental assistant writing a book for other fellow dental assistants?
   *I think it's incredibly valuable for dental assistants to learn about dental assisting from the perspective of a dentist because both parties will rely on mutual understanding while working together. The truth is there are few resources available that provide a broad perspective of dental assisting first-hand from dentists, and this reality inspired my writing. This book dismantles barriers and speculation for what dentists expect so dental assistants can establish and maintain a healthy working relationship within the dental team.*

# Index

**A**

Anesthetic 19, 38, 47, 52
Anterior 36, 37
Articulating paper 32,
    34, 38
Autoclave 26, 27, 28

**B**

Buccal 35, 37
Bur 32, 34, 38, 42

**C**

Cassette 27, 28, 29, 33,
    34, 38
Cavity 32, 41
Crown 42
Cure 32, 38
Curing 32
Curing light 31, 32, 38, 52

**D**

Dappen dish 32, 38, 52
Decay 32
Dental assisting 7
Dental hygienists 7
Dentin 32, 40
Desensitizer 31, 32, 38
Disinfection 26, 29
Distal 35, 37

**E**

Enamel 31, 32, 40
Ergonomics 44

**Etch** 31, 32, 38, 52
Etchant 31, 52
Explorer 32
Extraction 42

**F**

Facial 35, 37
Filling 30, 32, 38, 39
Four-handed Dentistry 7

**H**

Handpiece 33, 34, 38
High-volume suction 45

**I**

Impression 42
Incisal 35, 37
Infection control 26

**L**

Lingual 35, 37

**M**

Matrix 33, 38, 52
Mesial 35, 37
Modified pen grasp 46, 47

**O**

Occlusal 35, 37
Operatory 25, 26, 29, 30

**P**

Posterior 36, 37
Preparation 33
Prime and bond 33, 38, 52
Pulp 33, 43

**R**

Room turnover 26, 27
Root Canal 43

**S**

Shade 33
Shade Guide 33
Spray-wipe-spray 29
Sterilization 26, 27, 28, 29

**T**

Topical 33, 38, 52

**U**

Ultrasonic 27
Ultrasonic bath 26, 28

**V**

Vestibule 47

**W**

Wedge 33